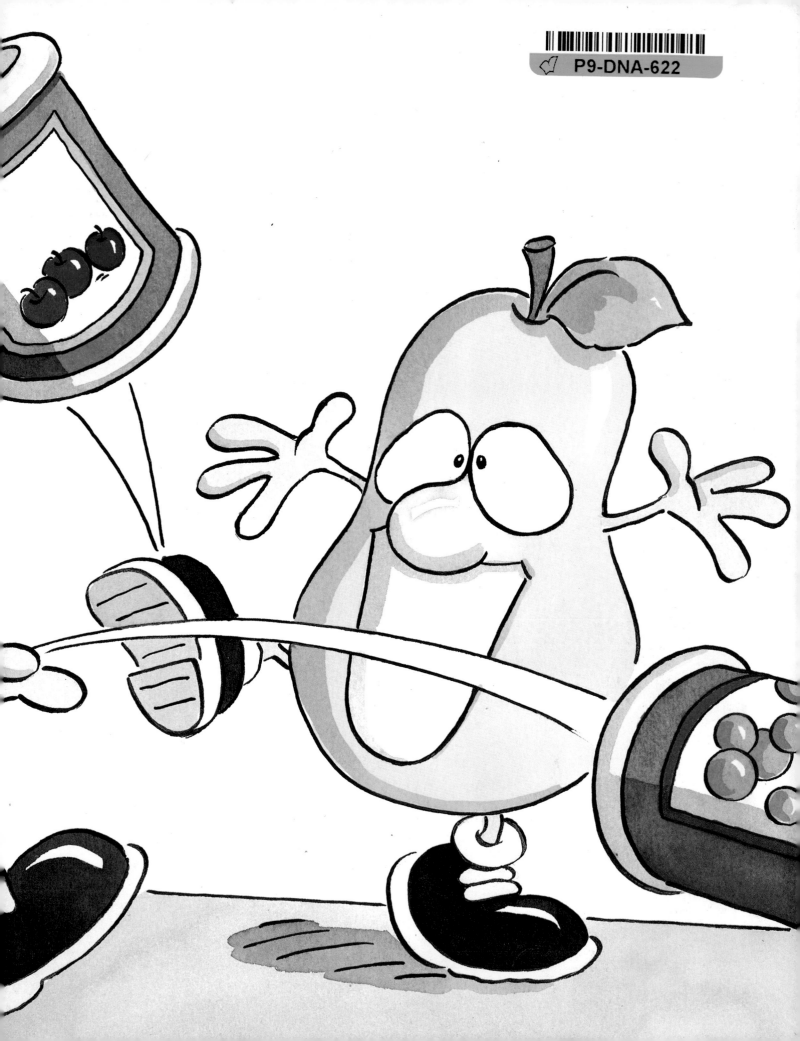

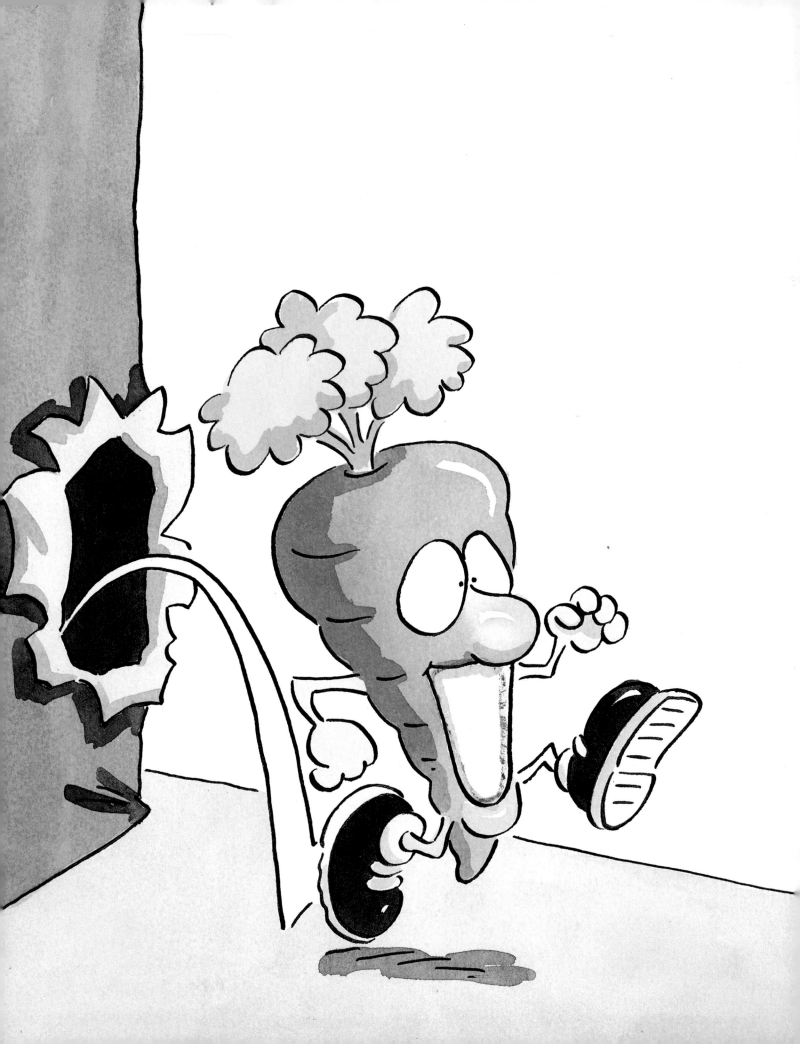

First Questions and Answers about **Food**

# What Makes Popcorn Pop?

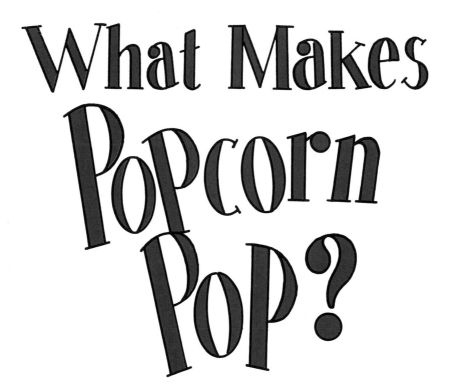

TIME LIFE for Children ®

ALEXANDRIA, VIRGINIA

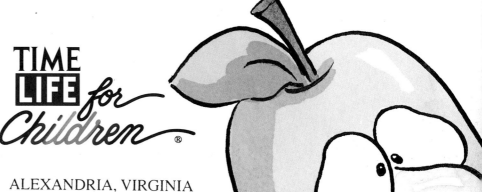

# Contents

Where does all the food come from?     4

Why do bananas have peels?     6

Where does orange juice come from?     8

Why are some foods in boxes and cans?     10

How are potato chips made?     12

Why do doughnuts have holes?     14

Where does chocolate come from?     16

Why do I have to wash fruits
and vegetables?     18

Can I still eat an apple
that turns brown?     20

Why do we keep some food cold?     22

Where does milk come from?     24

How do you make butter?     26

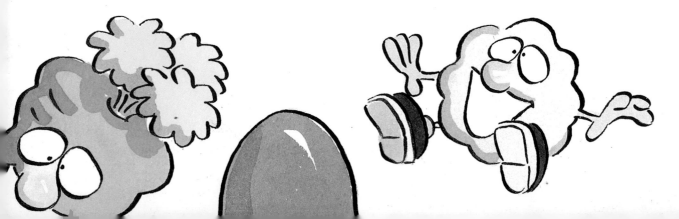

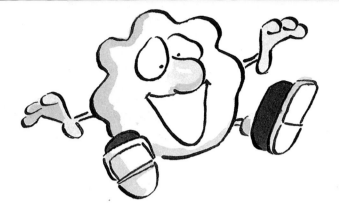

Is peanut butter made from butter? 28

How do you make bread? 30

Why does Swiss cheese have holes? 32

Where do raisins come from? 34

What makes popcorn pop? 36

Why does soda pop have bubbles? 38

Why is spaghetti hard before
  you cook it? 40

Why do I have to eat foods I don't like? 42

Where does pepper come from? 44

Do people eat the same food
  all around the world? 46

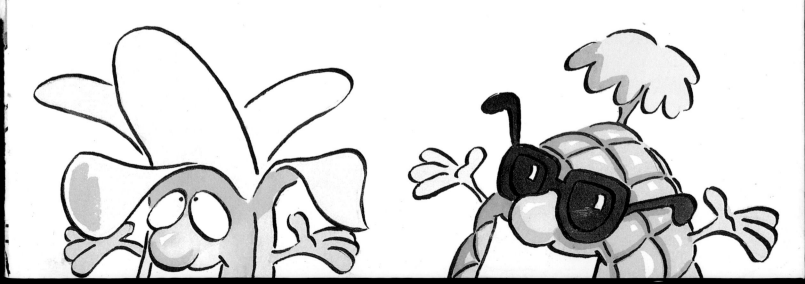

# Where does all the food come from?

Food in the grocery store comes from all over the world! It can come from very near your house or from thousands of miles away. Most food is grown on farms. Then it is carried in trains, planes, boats, or trucks to your neighborhood store.

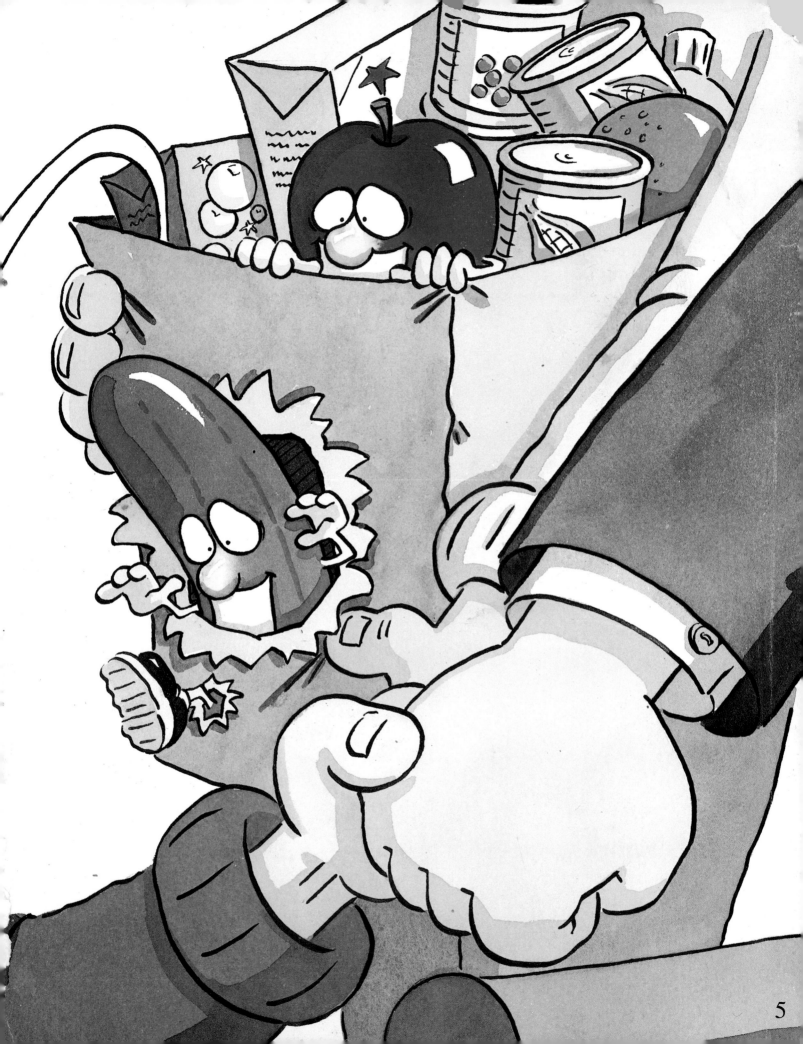

# Why do bananas have peels?

A banana's peel is its skin. The peel protects the banana inside. It keeps bugs from eating the banana. It also helps keep the soft fruit from freezing when it's cold out. If a banana gets cold, its skin will turn brown, but the fruit inside may still be white and tasty. Peel one and see!

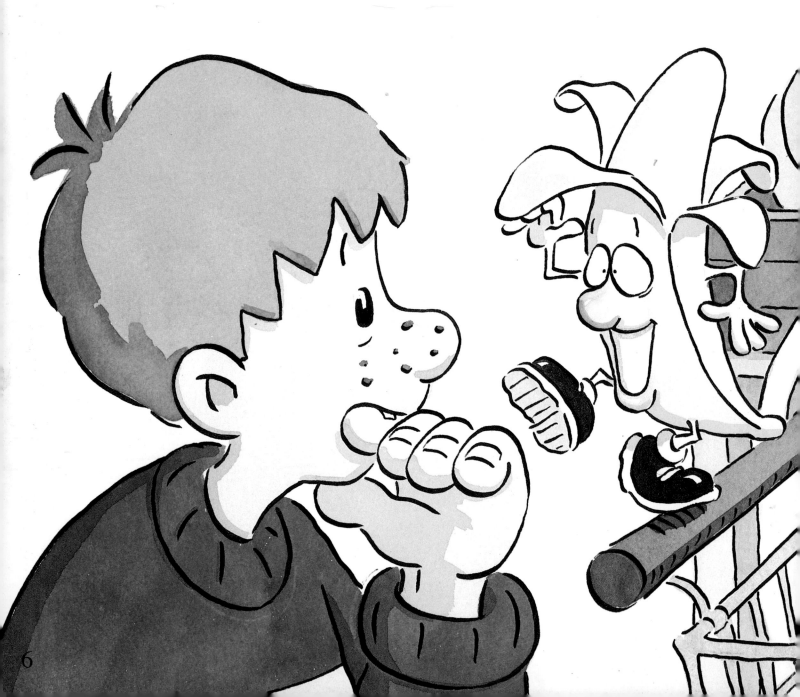

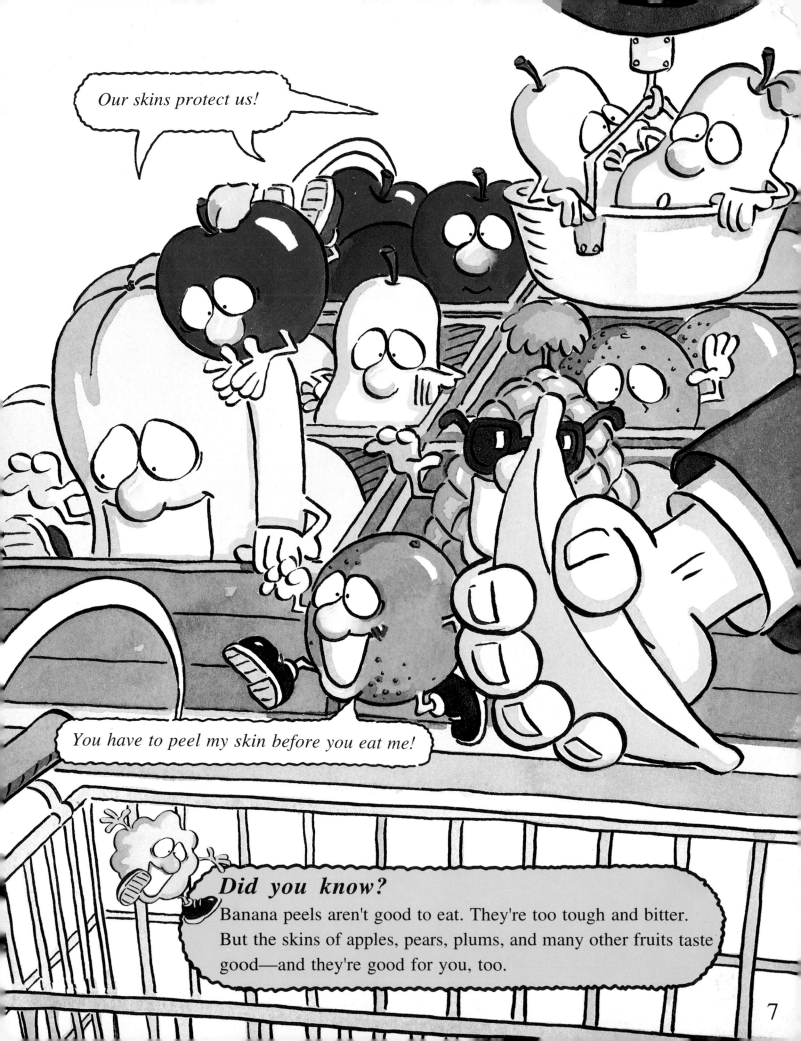

Did you know?
Banana peels aren't good to eat. They're too tough and bitter.
But the skins of apples, pears, plums, and many other fruits taste
good—and they're good for you, too.

# Where does orange juice come from?

Orange juice comes from oranges. Apple juice comes from apples. In fact, juice can be made from almost any fruit or vegetable—including carrots, grapes, lemons, and tomatoes.

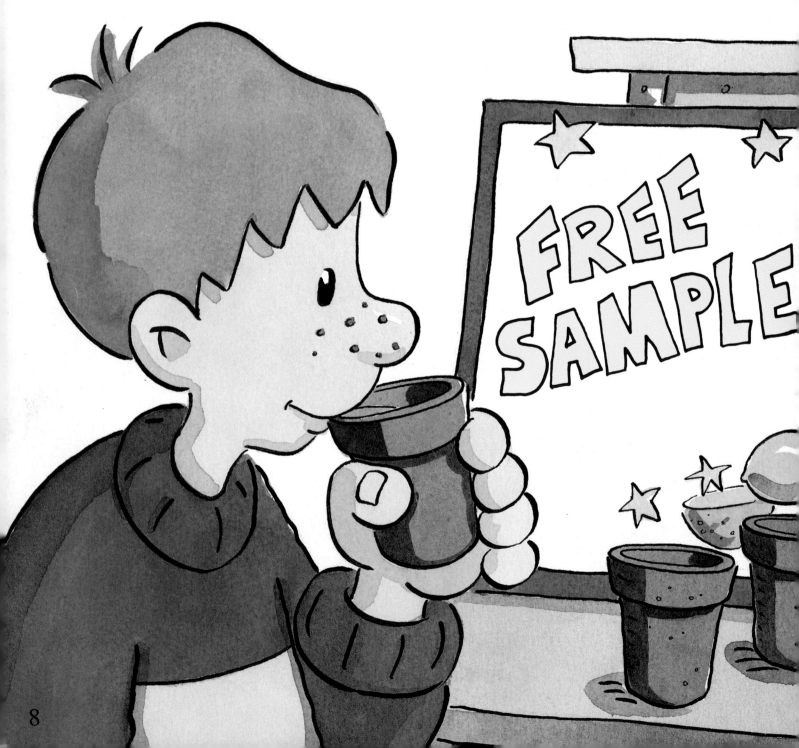

To make juice, the fruit or vegetable is cut up and then squeezed very hard. You can make juice at home, and some stores make their own juice. But most juice is made in factories, where big machines press the juice out of big piles of fruit all at once.

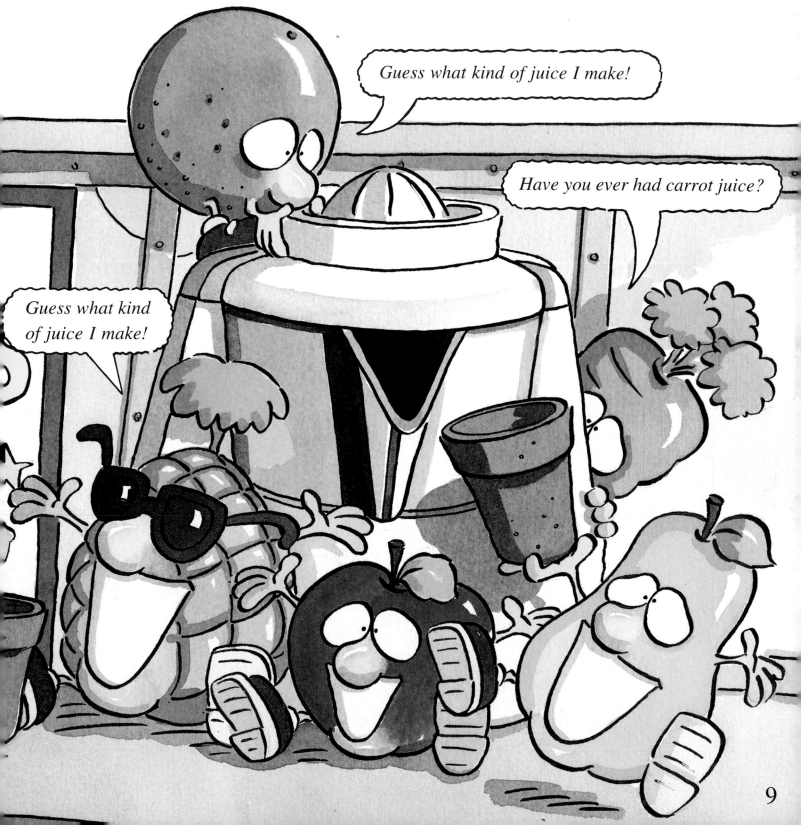

# Why are some foods in boxes and cans?

Because they last longer that way. Food that's put in a can lasts a long time. And boxes and bags keep food like cereal, potato chips, cookies, or crackers from getting crushed. We eat fresh fruit and vegetables right away, so they don't need to be packaged. But other foods stay on the shelf for a while, so they need special packages.

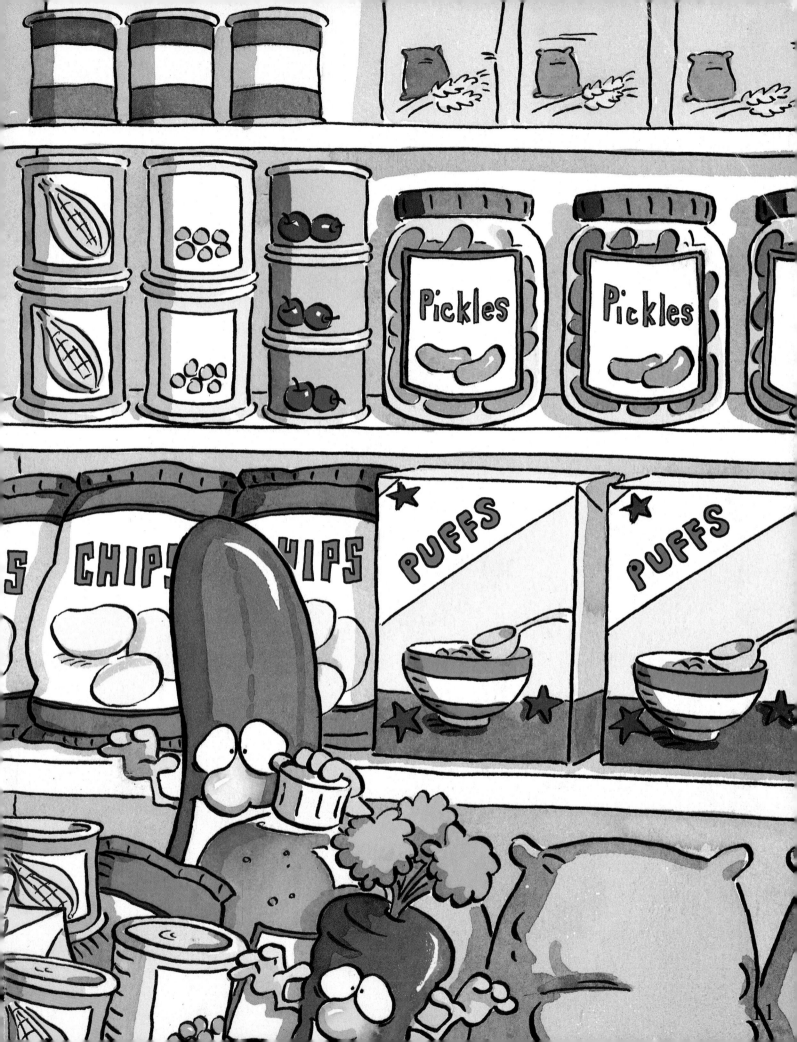

# How are potato chips made?

Potato chips are made from potatoes.

**Did you know?**
French fries are made from potatoes that are cut into bigger pieces before they are cooked. French fries get crispy on the outside but stay soft inside.

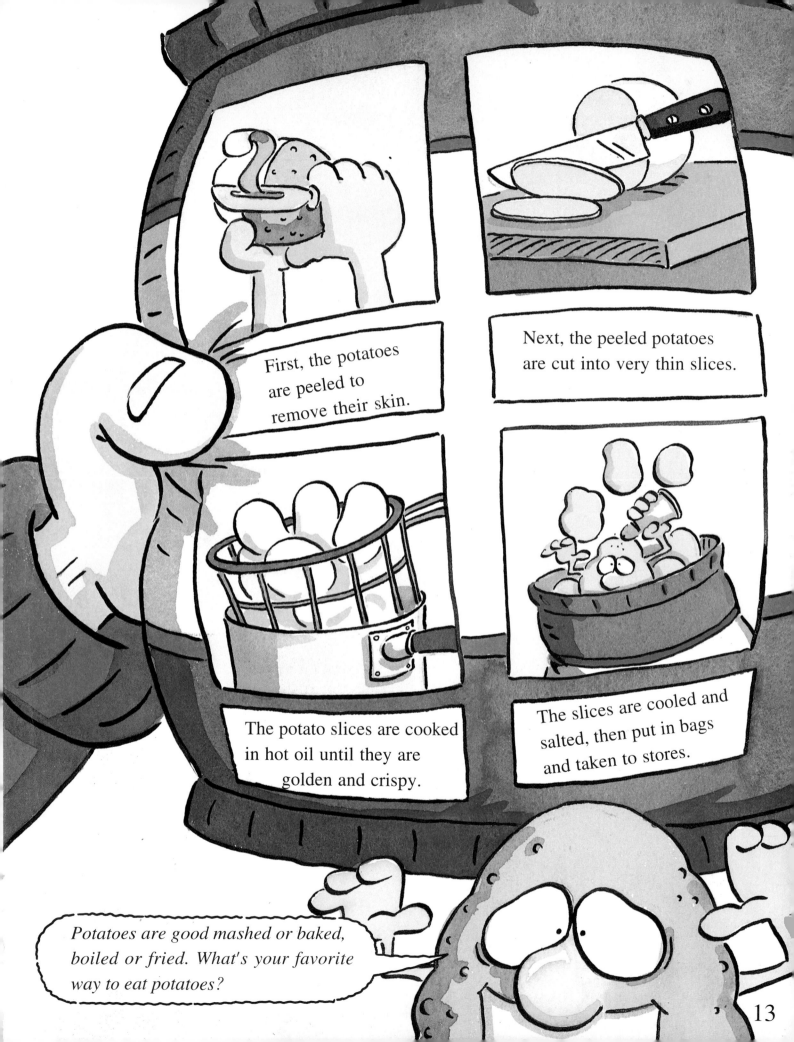

First, the potatoes are peeled to remove their skin.

Next, the peeled potatoes are cut into very thin slices.

The potato slices are cooked in hot oil until they are golden and crispy.

The slices are cooled and salted, then put in bags and taken to stores.

*Potatoes are good mashed or baked, boiled or fried. What's your favorite way to eat potatoes?*

# Why do doughnuts have holes?

Doughnuts are made from sweet dough fried in hot oil. A long time ago, doughnuts didn't have holes, so their insides didn't cook when they were fried. Then a little boy had a very good idea: If the middle doesn't cook, take it out! His mother cut out the center, and the doughnuts cooked perfectly. Ever since then, people have been making doughnuts with holes.

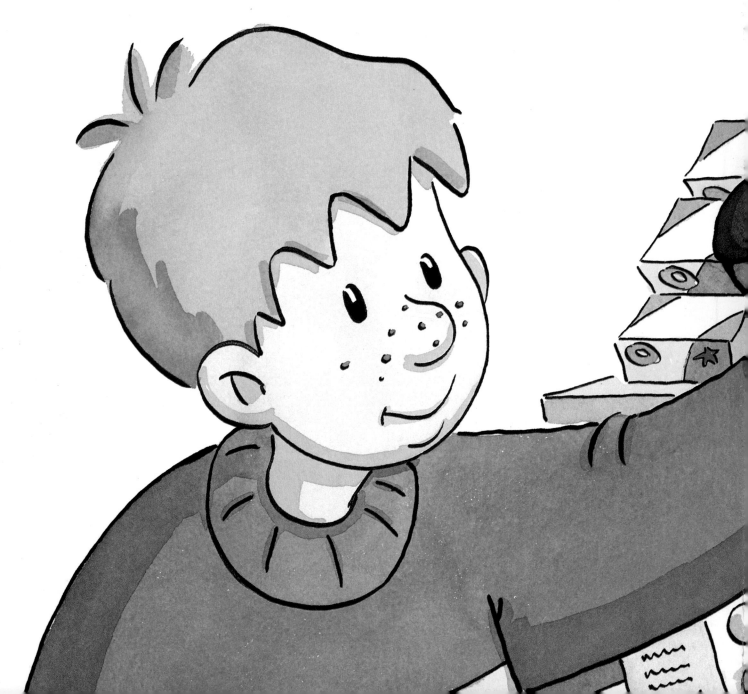

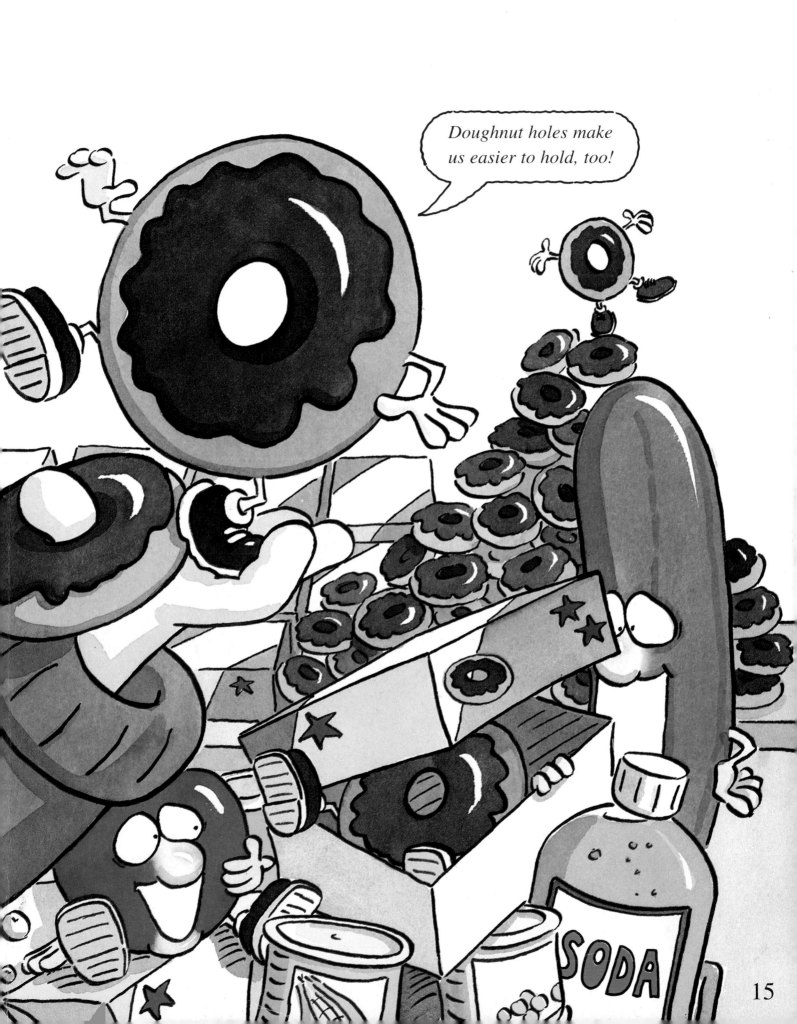

15

# Where does chocolate come from?

Chocolate is made from cocoa beans. Cocoa beans grow on trees in countries that are very far away.

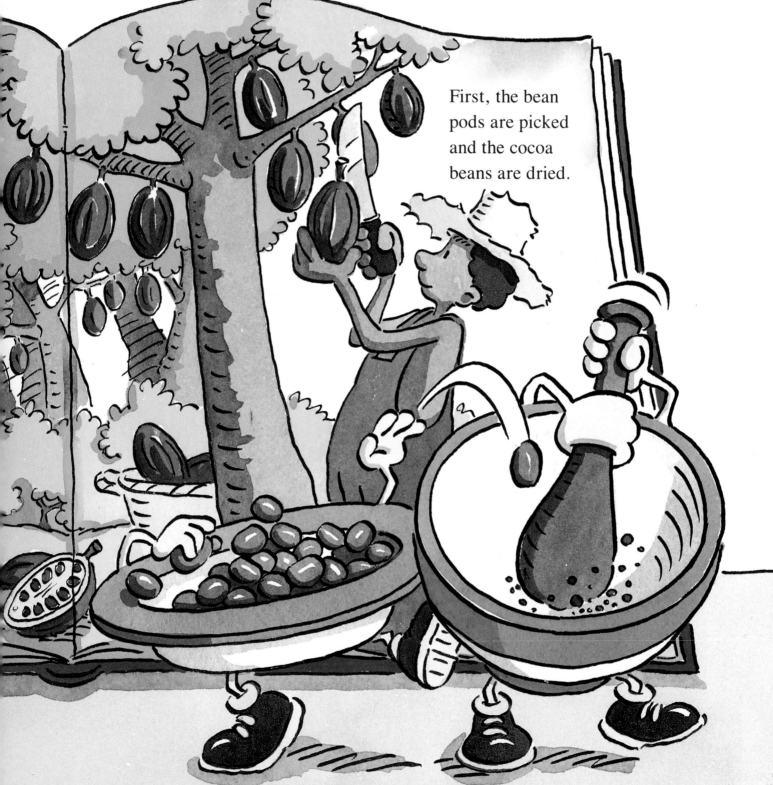

First, the bean pods are picked and the cocoa beans are dried.

Next, the dried beans are cooked and ground up to make cocoa.

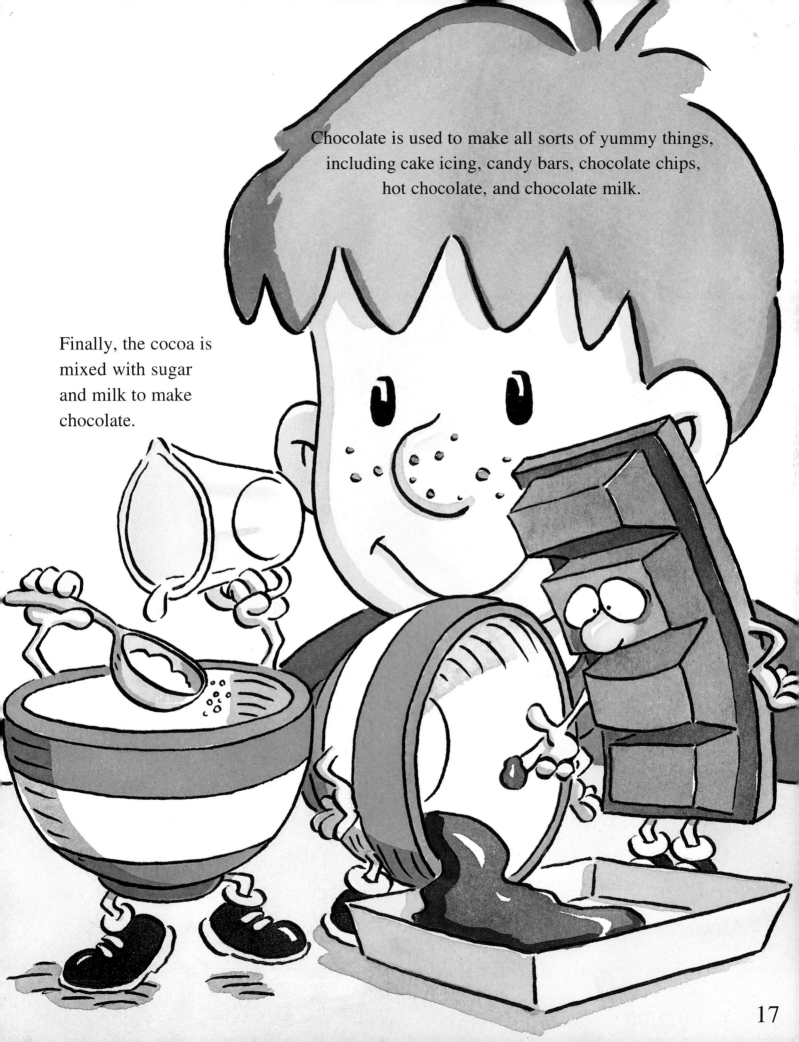

Chocolate is used to make all sorts of yummy things, including cake icing, candy bars, chocolate chips, hot chocolate, and chocolate milk.

Finally, the cocoa is mixed with sugar and milk to make chocolate.

# Why do I have to wash fruits and vegetables?

Because they might have dirt on them. Farmers grow the fruits and vegetables. But they don't want bugs to eat the food before it gets to the store, so they spray it with something that keeps the bugs away. This spray protects the food, but it isn't good for you to eat. It needs to be scrubbed off.

*I may look clean, but I need to be washed, too.*

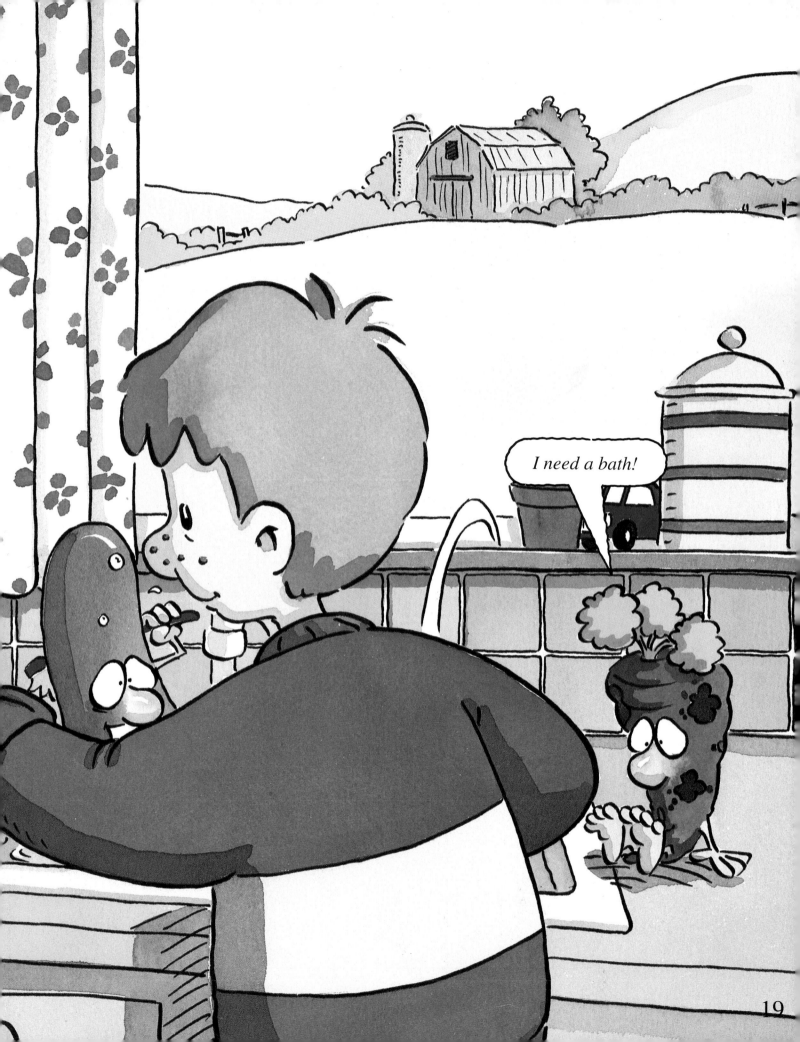

19

# Can I still eat an apple that turns brown?

Yes. Apples begin to turn brown as soon as you bite them. But the brown isn't bad. When air touches an apple after its skin comes off, the air mixes with the fruit inside to turn it brown. This is the apple's way of making a new skin, which protects it just like the old one.

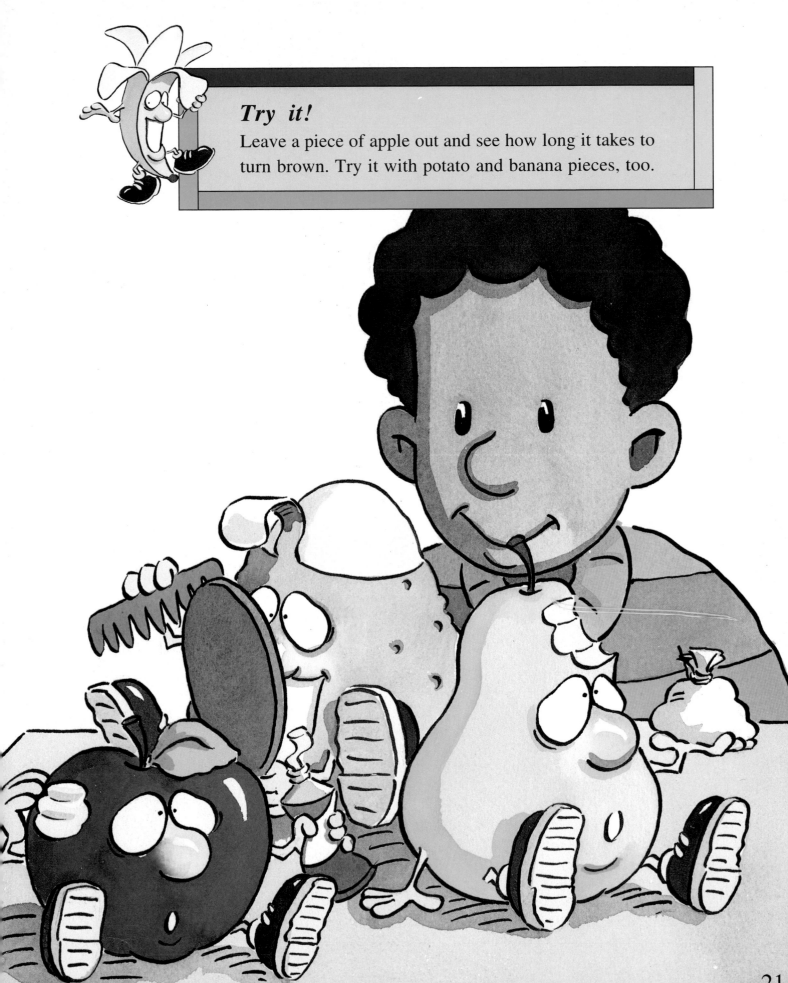

21

# Why do we keep some food cold?

Some foods spoil when they are kept in warm air. But in the cold air inside a refrigerator, these foods stay fresh for a long time. Another way to keep food from spoiling is to freeze it. Ice cream will melt unless it stays frozen.

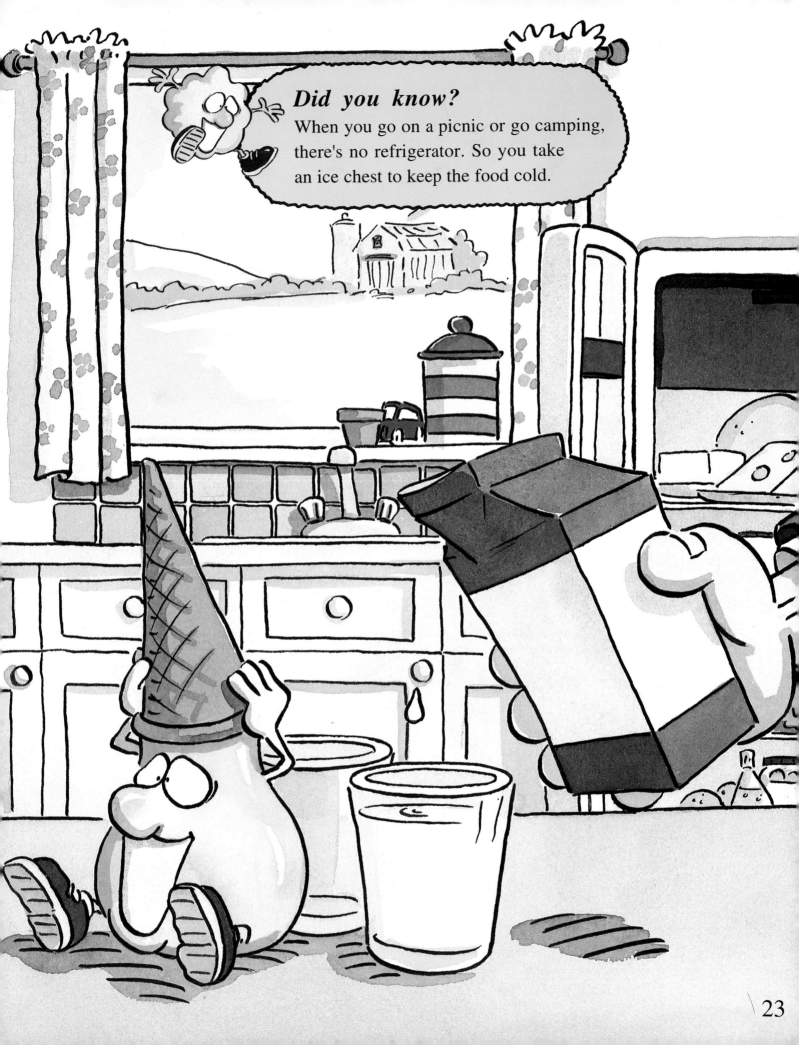

**Did you know?**
When you go on a picnic or go camping, there's no refrigerator. So you take an ice chest to keep the food cold.

# Where does milk come from?

Before it gets put into containers and sold at supermarkets, most milk comes from cows. Cows make milk for their babies, called calves. When the calves are older, farmers milk cows by squeezing their udders. A cow needs to be milked in the morning and at night. One cow can make enough milk in one day to fill 160 glasses!

*Did you know?*
People drink milk from goats, buffalo, camels, and reindeers as well as cows. Foods made from milk, such as butter, cheese, and yogurt, are called dairy products.

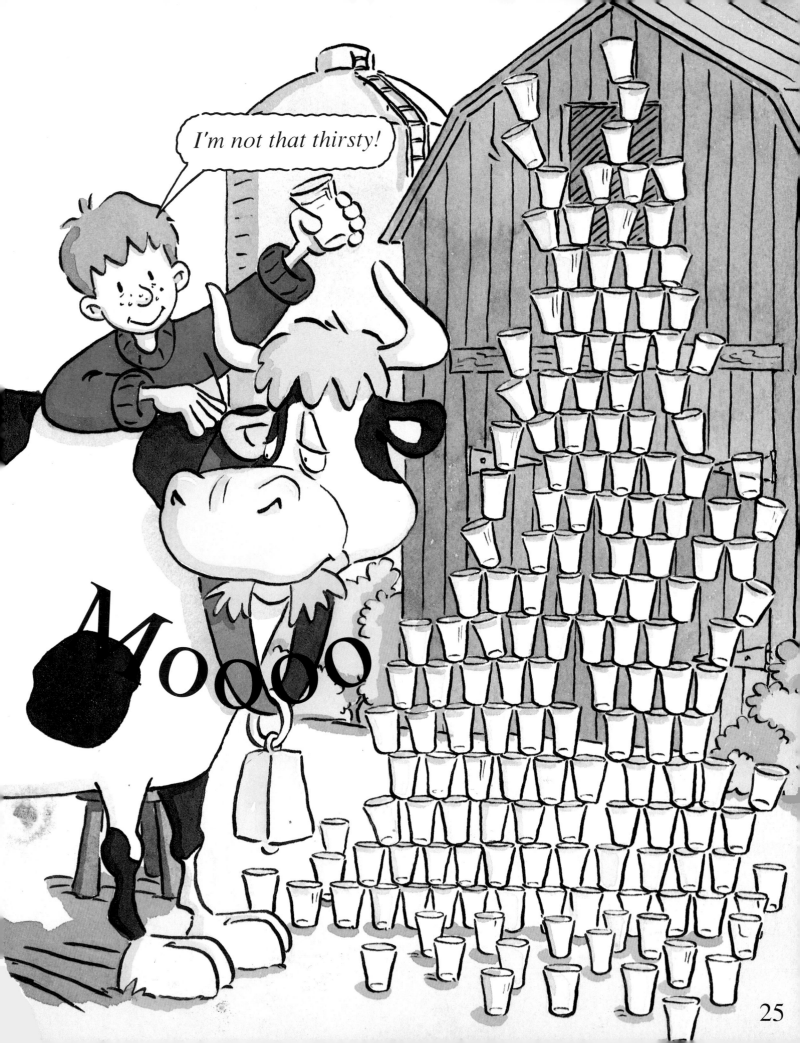

# How do you make butter?

Butter is made from cream. The milk that comes out of a cow has thick, heavy cream floating on top. This is usually skimmed off and put in a different carton. Some cream, though, is stirred over and over again. Another word for this stirring is churning. The cream is churned until big chunks of butter float to the top. These chunks are molded into sticks or packed into tubs and sent to the store.

**Try it!**

With a parent's help, you can make butter at home. Pour some heavy cream into a plastic container with a tight-fitting lid. Then start shaking the container. After about 10 minutes of shaking, chunks of butter will appear.

# Is peanut butter made from butter?

No, peanut butter is made from crushed peanuts. Peanuts are cooked and then ground together until they form creamy, thick peanut butter. Some kinds of peanut butter have sugar, salt, and oil mixed in, too. We call it peanut butter because it spreads on bread and other foods the same way butter does.

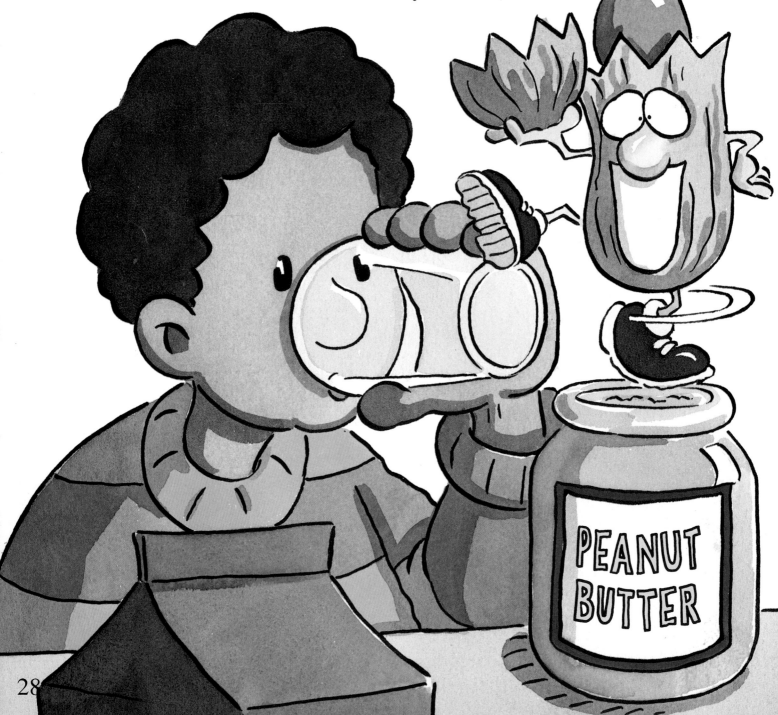

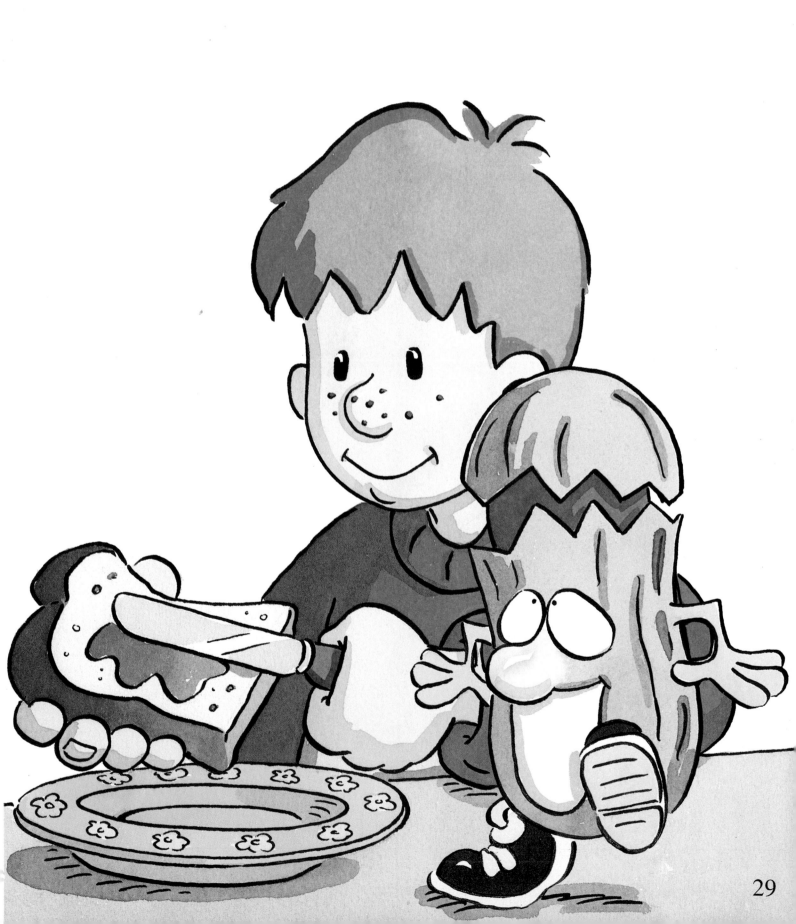

# How do you make bread?

Bread comes in many different shapes, sizes, flavors, and colors. But almost all bread is made from flour and water.

**Try it!**
Look carefully at a piece of bread. Can you see the tiny bubbles made by the yeast?

First, the flour and water are mixed to make dough. Sometimes salt or sugar is added to the dough. Most bread also has yeast in it. Yeast looks like small grains of sand.

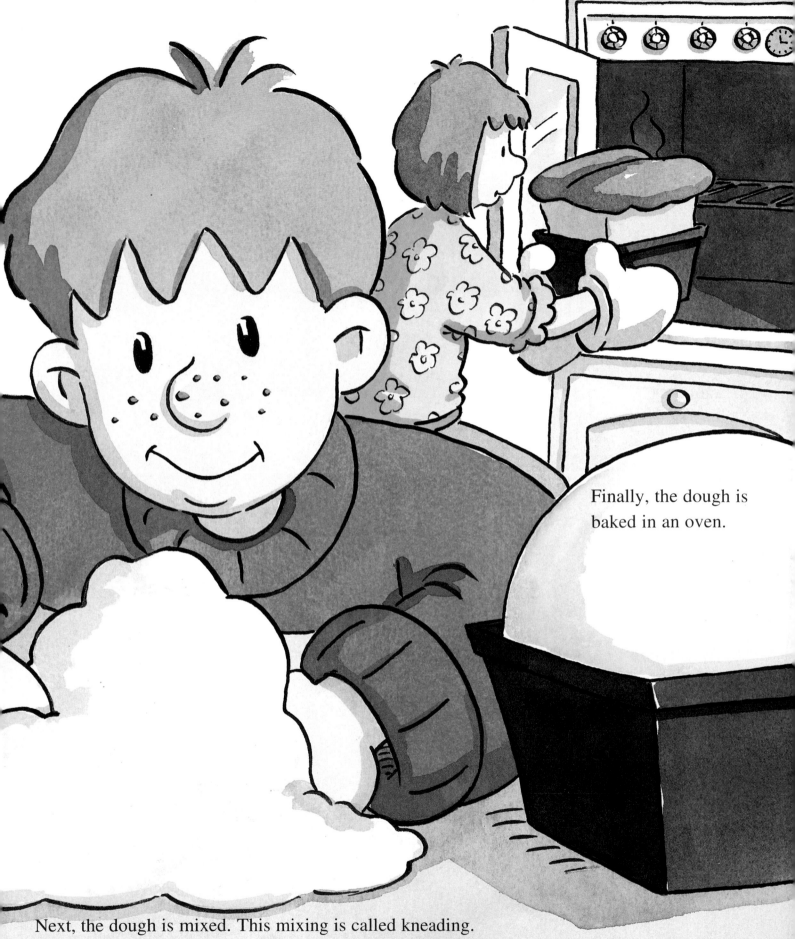

Finally, the dough is baked in an oven.

Next, the dough is mixed. This mixing is called kneading.
Then the dough is left to sit for a while to rise, or get bigger.
The dough rises because the yeast bubbles up inside it.

3

# Why does Swiss cheese have holes?

The holes are from bubbles that pop when the cheese is being made. Like butter and ice cream, Swiss cheese starts out as milk. The milk is heated, and different things are added. Then the mixture is left to turn slowly into cheese. While it sits, bubbles form. Every bubble leaves a hole.

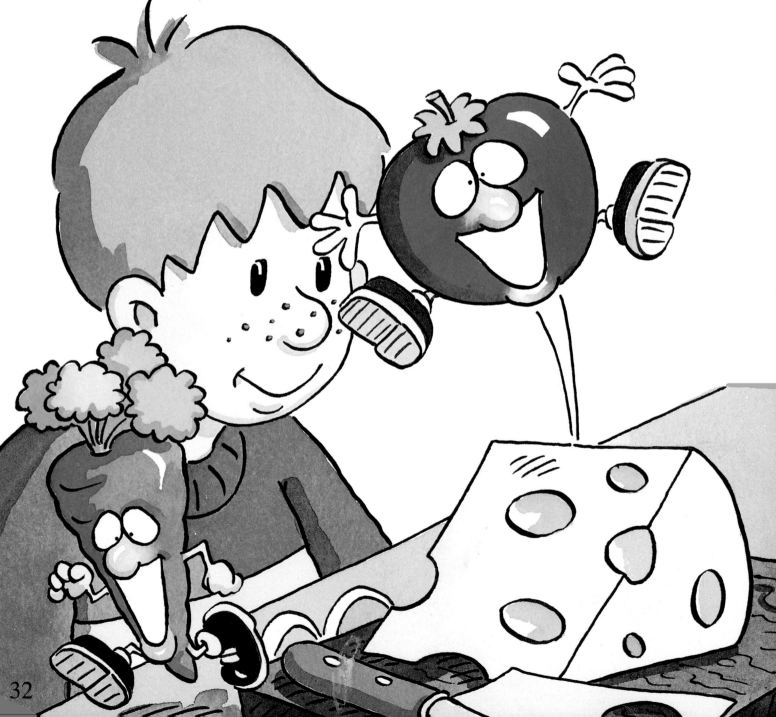

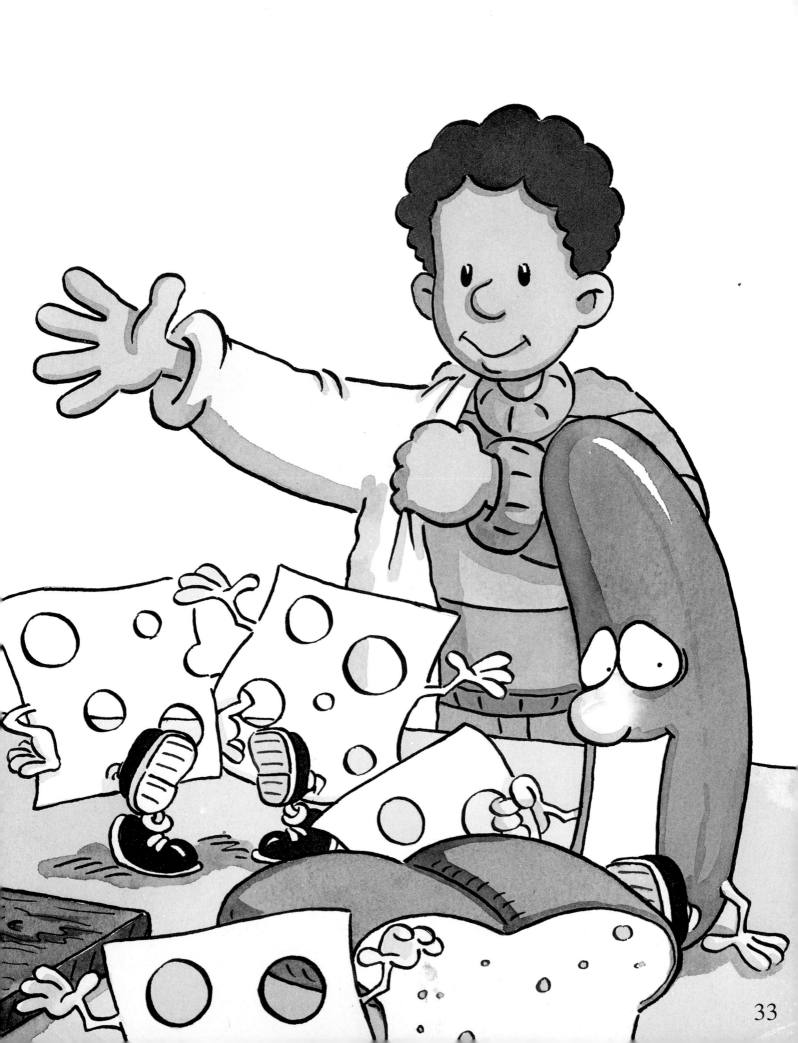

# Where do raisins come from?

Raisins are made from grapes! After the grapes are picked, they are dried in the sun. As they dry, they darken and shrivel up, getting smaller and smaller. Then the raisins are washed, packed in boxes, and shipped to your store.

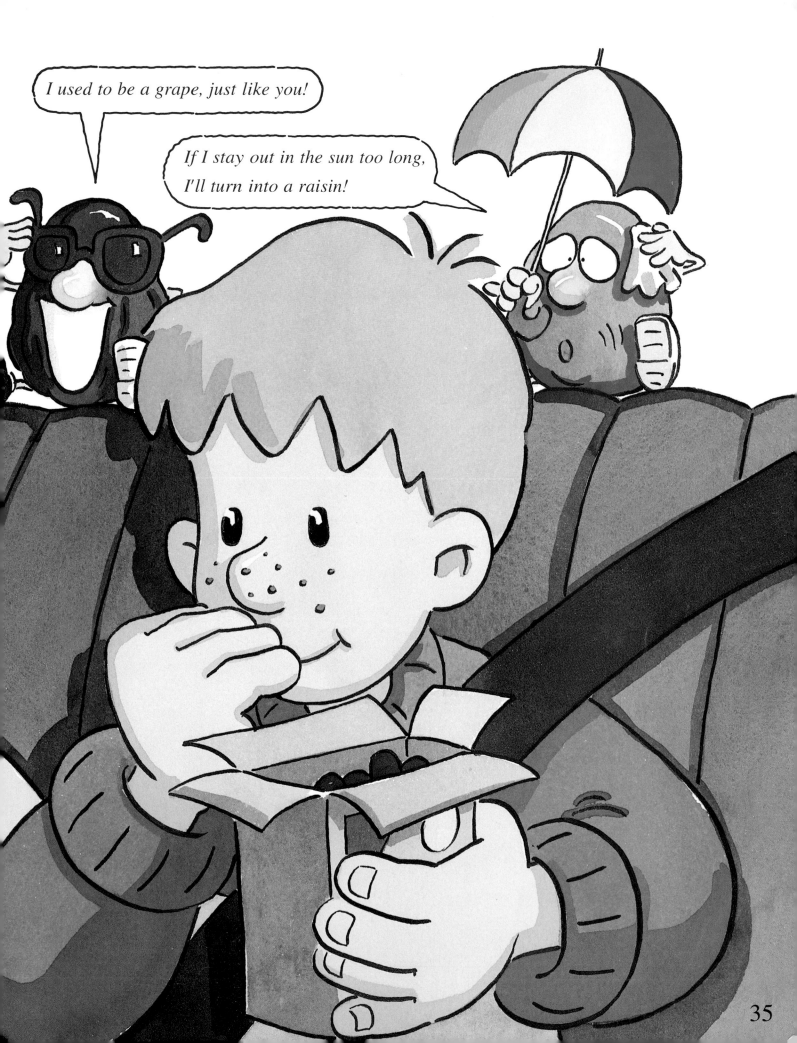

# What makes popcorn pop?

A piece of unpopped popcorn is called a kernel. Every popcorn kernel has water inside it. When the kernel is heated, the water gets hot and boils, just like water in a kettle on the stove. The boiling water bursts through the kernel's outer skin, and the kernel explodes with a great big "POP!"

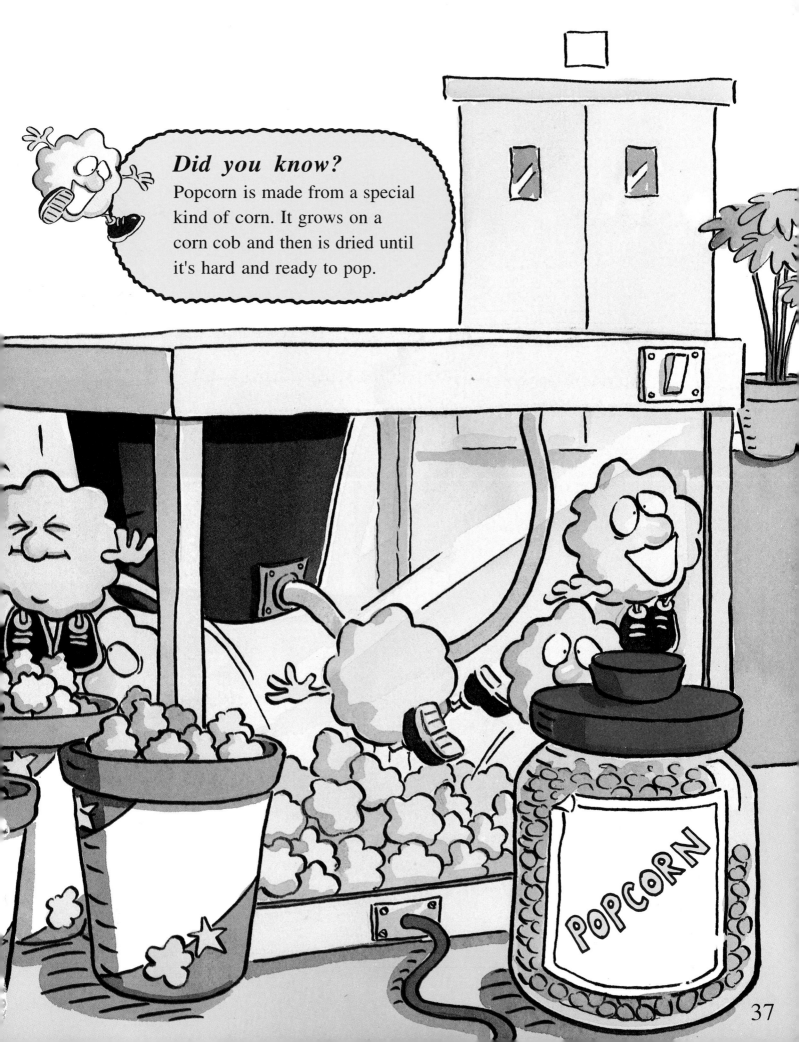

**Did you know?**
Popcorn is made from a special kind of corn. It grows on a corn cob and then is dried until it's hard and ready to pop.

# Why does soda pop have bubbles?

Soda pop starts out as a sweet drink with no fizz. Then bubbles are blown into a can or bottle, and it's closed tightly with the bubbles inside. When the can is opened, the bubbles try to rush out all at once. Ps-s-h-ht!

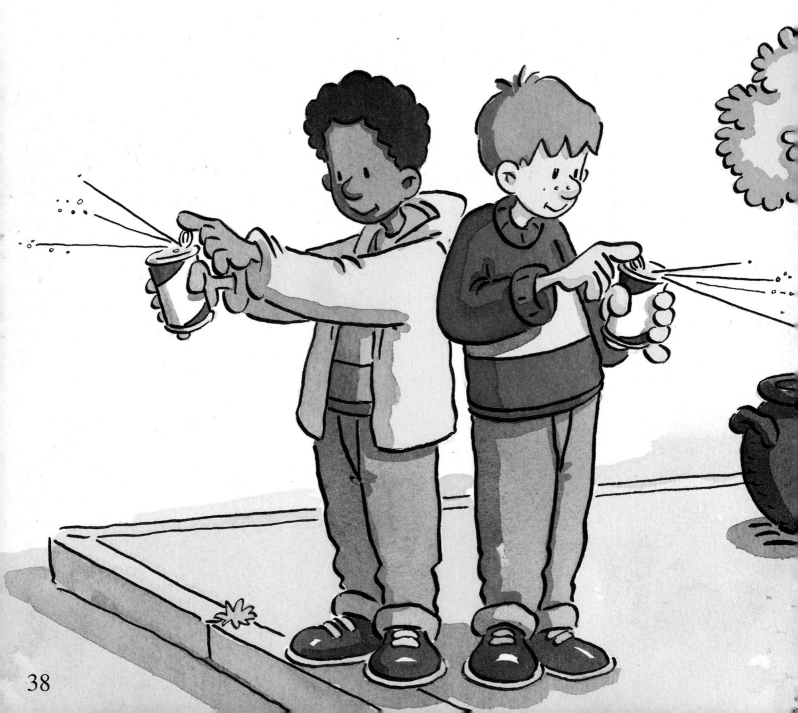

POTS OF PASTA

TODAY'S SPECIALS

# Why is spaghetti hard before you cook it?

Spaghetti starts out as soft dough made of flour and water. The dough is pushed through tiny holes and comes out as long, soft strings. The spaghetti strings are left to dry, which takes the water out and makes them hard. When the spaghetti is cooked, the water goes back in and makes it soft again.

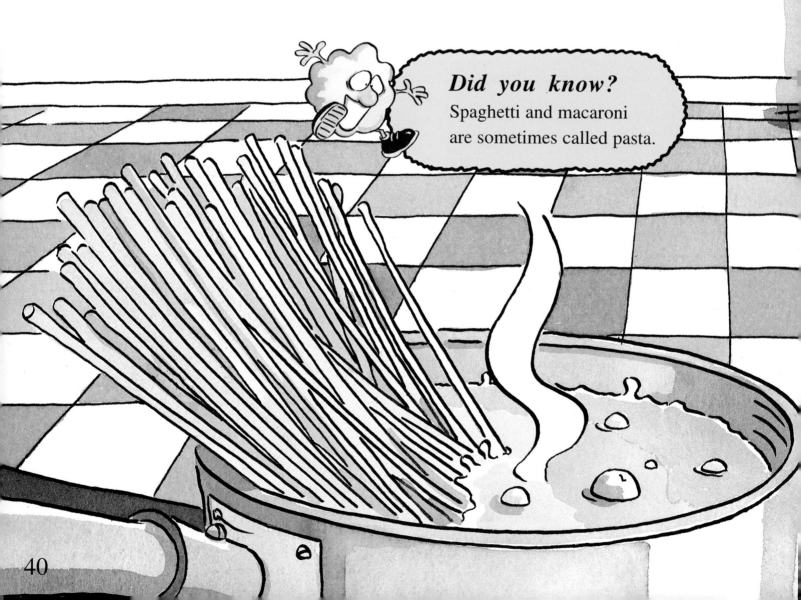

**Did you know?**
Spaghetti and macaroni are sometimes called pasta.

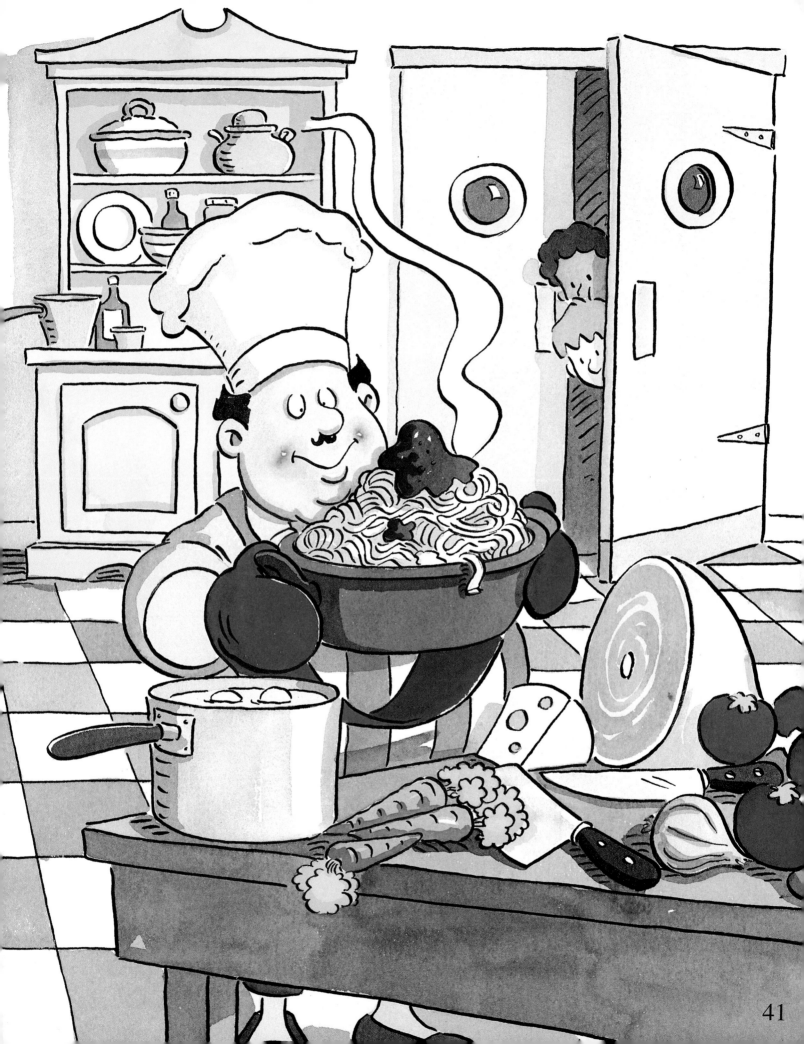

# Why do I have to eat foods I don't like?

Sometimes you have to eat foods you don't like because they're good for you. Everyone needs to eat different kinds of food to stay healthy.

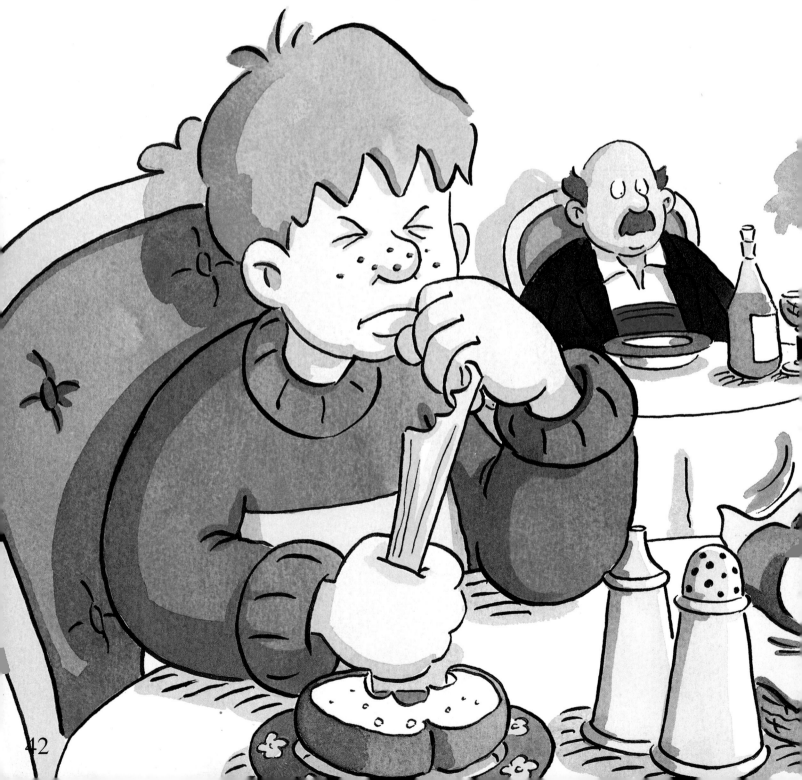

Each kind of food has something in it that you need. Even though you don't like a food now, your tastes will change. You may love a food tomorrow that you dislike today. So it's important to keep trying new foods. One of them may turn out to be your favorite!

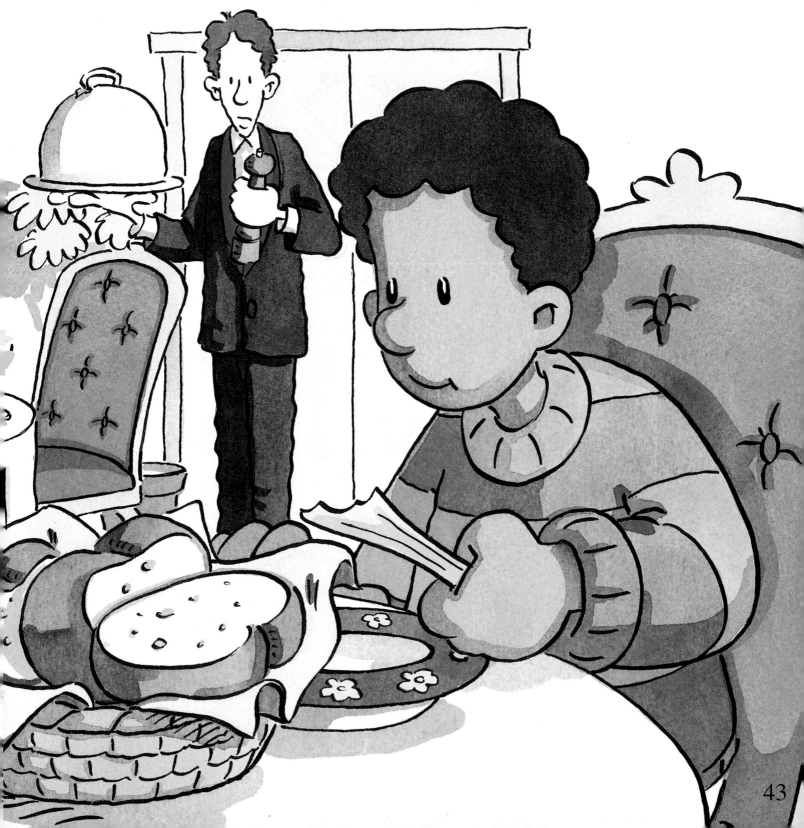

# Where does pepper come from?

The pepper we put on food comes from red berries that are dried in the sun until they turn black. These round black peppercorns are ground up to make pepper. Pepper makes food tasty, but don't sniff it—it will make you sneeze. Ah-Choo!

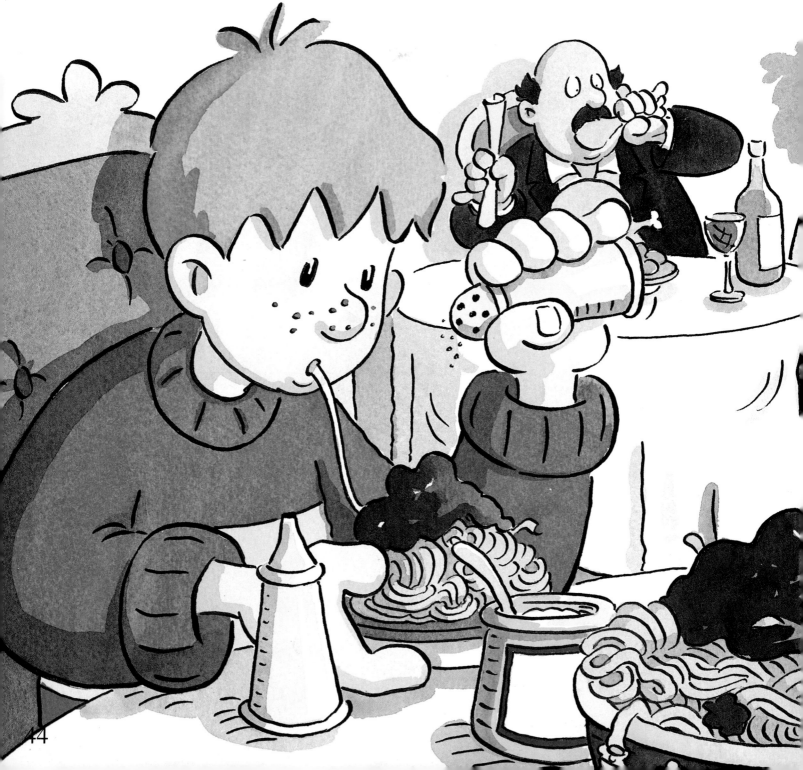

**Did you know?**
Most salt comes from the ocean or from beneath the ground. Salt makes food taste good, but too much salt is bad for you.

45

# Do people eat the same food all around the world?

Everyone all over the world eats pretty much the same kinds of food that you do: milk and cheese, vegetables and fruit, meat and fish, bread, pasta, and rice. But different people cook food in different ways, and people in different parts of the world use different spices, so the food tastes different.

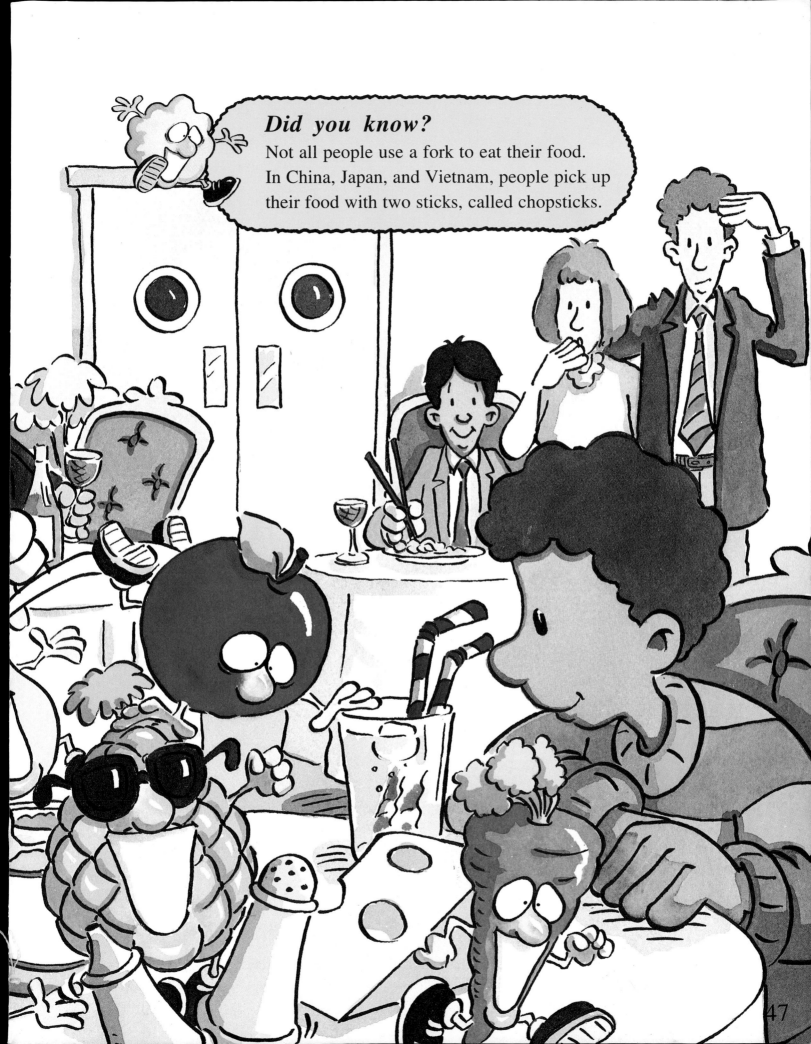

**Did you know?**
Not all people use a fork to eat their food. In China, Japan, and Vietnam, people pick up their food with two sticks, called chopsticks.

47

**TIME-LIFE for CHILDREN** ®

**Managing Editor:** Patricia Daniels
**Editorial Directors:** Jean Burke Crawford, Allan Fallow,
                                        Karin Kinney, Sara Mark, Elizabeth Ward
**Publishing Assistant:** Marike van der Veen
**Production Manager:** Marlene Zack
**Senior Copyeditor:** Colette Stockum
**Production:** Celia Beattie
**Supervisor of Quality Control:** James King
**Assistant Supervisor of Quality Control:** Miriam Newton
**Library:** Louise D. Forstall, Anne Heising

**Special Contributor:** Barbara Klein
**Researcher:** Eugenia Scharf
**Writer:** Jacqueline A. Ball

| | |
|---|---|
| **Designed by:** | **David Bennett Books** |
| **Series design:** | David Bennett |
| **Book design:** | Andrew Crowson |
| **Art direction:** | David Bennett & Andrew Crowson |
| **Illustrated by:** | Andy Cooke |
| **Additional cover** | |
| **illustrations by:** | Malcolm Livingstone |

First printing. Printed in U.S.A.
Published simultaneously in Canada.

Time Life Inc. is a wholly owned subsidiary of THE TIME INC. BOOK COMPANY.

TIME-LIFE is a trademark of Time Warner Inc. U.S.A.

For subscription information, call 1-800-621-7026.

**Library of Congress Cataloging-in-Publication Data**

What makes popcorn pop?: first questions and answers about food.
        p.  cm. -- (Time-Life library of first questions and answers)
        ISBN 0-7835-0862-X. -- ISBN 0-7835-0863-8 (lib. bdg.)
    1. Food--Miscellanea--Juvenile literature.  2. Diet--Miscellanea--Juvenile literature.  [1. Food--Miscellanea.  2.
    Questions and answers.]  I. Time-Life for Children (Firm)  II. Series: Library of first questions and answers.
TX355.W43  1994
641.3--dc20
                                                                                    93-28880
                                                                                        CIP
                                                                                         AC

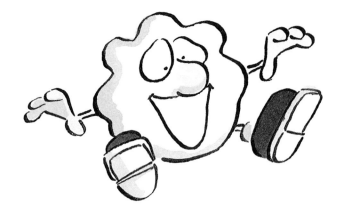

**Consultants**

**Dr. Lewis P. Lipsitt**, an internationally recognized specialist on childhood
development, was the 1990 recipient of the Nicholas Hobbs Award for science in the
service of children. He has served as the science director for the American
Psychological Association and is a professor of psychology and medical science at
Brown University.

**Dr. Judith A. Schickedanz**, an authority on the education of preschool children, is
an associate professor of early childhood education at the Boston University School
of Education, where she also directs the Early Childhood Learning Laboratory. Her
published work includes *More Than the ABC's: Early Stages of Reading and Writing
Development* as well as several textbooks and many scholarly papers.

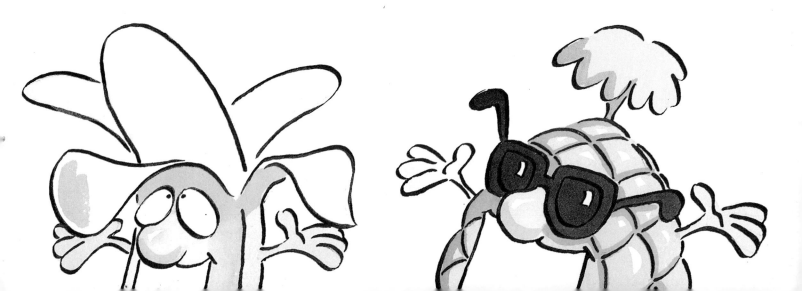

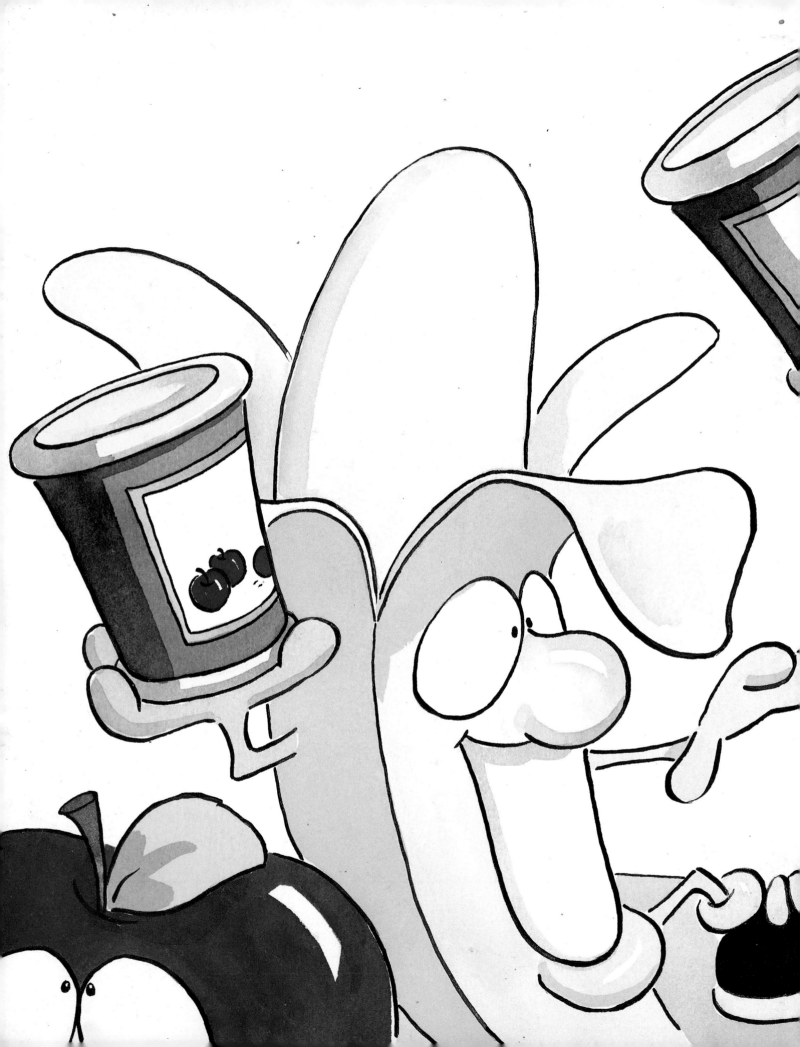